Vibrant Anti Inflammatory Diet Cookbook

Quick and Easy Breakfast Recipes for Beginners

Zac Gibson

Table of Contents

Bacon and Egg Breakfast Chili

Prep Time:
25 minutes
Serve: 8

Ingredients:
- 1 pound of breakfast sausage, thawed and roughly chopped
- ½ pound of bacon, chopped
- 6 large organic eggs
- 1 medium white onion, finely chopped
- 2 tablespoons of olive oil
- 1 (28-ounce can of diced tomatoes with green chiles 2-3 cups of homemade low-sodium chicken broth
- 2 teaspoons of smoked paprika or regular paprika
- 2 teaspoons of chili powder
- 2 teaspoons of garlic powder
- 1 teaspoon of onion powder
- 1 teaspoon of fine sea salt Avocado slices

Directions:

1.Press the "Sauté" function on your Instant Pot and add the bacon. Cook until brown and crispy, stirring occasionally.

2.Transfer the bacon to a plate lined with paper towels.

3.Add the breakfast sausage and onions to the bacon grease and cook until the sausage has browned.

4.Add the remaining ingredients except for the eggs to your

5.Instant Pot. Lock the lid and cook at high pressure for 10 minutes.

6.When the cooking is done, naturally release the pressure and remove the lid

7.Meanwhile, fry or scramble your eggs on a stovetop skillet the way you like.

8.You can skip this step if you only want to use your Instant Pot.

9.Once everything is done, scoop the breakfast chili onto bowls and top with eggs, bacon, and avocado slices.

Nutrition: Calories: 441, Fat: 34.9g, Net Carb: 3.4g, Protein: 26.5g

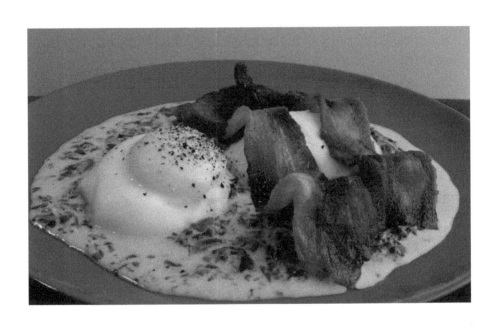

Lemon Blueberry Muffin

Prep Time:
15 minutes
Serve: 6

Ingredients:
- 2 cups of almond flour
- 1 cup of heavy whipping cream
- 2 large organic eggs, beaten
- ¼ cup of coconut butter or ghee, melt
- 1 tablespoon of granulated erythritol or other keto-friendly sweeteners
- ½ cup of fresh or frozen blueberries
- 1 teaspoon of fresh lemon zest
- 1 teaspoon of lemon extract
- 1/8 teaspoon of fine sea salt

Directions:

1.In a large bowl, add all the ingredients and gently stir until well combined.

2.Grease 6 silicone muffin cups with nonstick cooking spray
Divide and add the muffin batter into each muffin cup.

3.Add 1 cup of water and a trivet inside your Instant Pot. Place the muffin cup on top of the trivet and cover with aluminum foil.

4.Lock the lid and cook at high pressure for 8 minutes. When the timer beeps, naturally release the pressure for 10 minutes. Carefully remove the lid.

5.Check if the muffins are cooked by using a toothpick.

Nutrition: Calories: 220, Fat: 21g, Net Carb: 3g, Protein: 4g

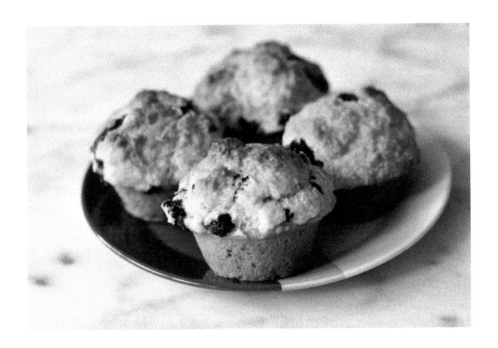

Zucchini Muffins

Prep Time:
15 minutes
Serve: 6

Ingredients:

- 1 large zucchini, finely grated
- 6 medium bacon slices, chopped
- 4 large organic eggs
- ½ cup of heavy whipping cream
- 1 cup of shredded cheddar cheese
- 1 cup of almond flour
- 4 tablespoons of flax meal
- ½ cup of parmesan cheese, finely grated
- 1 tablespoon of dried Italian herbs
- 2 teaspoons of onion powder
- 1 teaspoon of baking powder
- ½ teaspoon of garlic powder
- ½ teaspoon of fine sea salt
- ½ teaspoon of freshly cracked black pepper

Directions:

1.Grease 6 silicone muffin cups with nonstick cooking spray.

2.In a large bowl, add all the ingredients and gently stir until well combined.

3.Divide and spoon the batter into each muffin cup.

4.Add 2 cups of water and a trivet inside your Instant Pot. Place the muffin cups on top and cover with aluminum foil.

5.Lock the lid and cook at high pressure for 10 minutes. When the cooking is done, naturally release the pressure for 10 minutes. Carefully remove the lid and check if the muffins are done.

Nutrition: Calories: 216, Fat: 17g, Net Carb: 2.7g, Protein: 12.9g

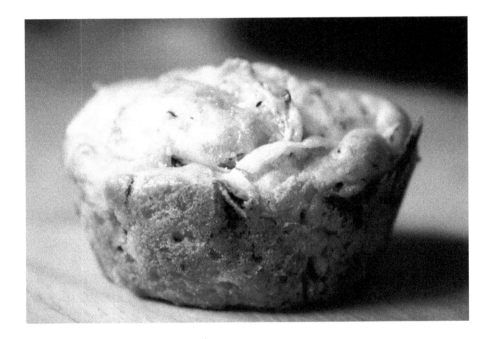

Italian Sausage Breakfast Cups

Prep Time:
20 minutes
Serve: 4

Ingredients:

- 1 pound of Italian sausage links, cut into bite-sized pieces
- 4 large eggs, beaten
- 1 medium yellow or white onion, finely chopped
- 1 teaspoon of fine sea salt
- 1 teaspoon of freshly cracked black pepper
- ½ cup of mushrooms, finely chopped
- ½ cup of broccoli florets, chopped
- ½ cup of spinach, roughly chopped
- 1 tablespoon of fresh parsley, finely chopped
- 2 tablespoons of olive oil

Directions:

1.Press the "Sauté" function on your Instant Pot and add the olive oil. Once hot, add the onions, mushrooms, and broccoli. Cook until softened, stirring occasionally. Remove and set aside.

2.Add the Italian sausage and cook until brown, stirring occasionally. Turn off "Sauté" function on your Instant Pot.

3.In a large bowl, add the vegetables, cooked Italian sausage and remaining ingredients. Stir until well combined. Divide the mixture between 6 silicon muffin cups or greased ramekins.

4.Add 1 cup of water and a trivet inside your Instant Pot. Place the muffin cups on top and lock the lid. Cook at high pressure for 10 minutes.

5.When the cooking is done, naturally release the pressure and carefully remove the lid.

Nutrition: Calories: 288, Fat: 23g, Net Carb: 1g, Protein: 16.5g

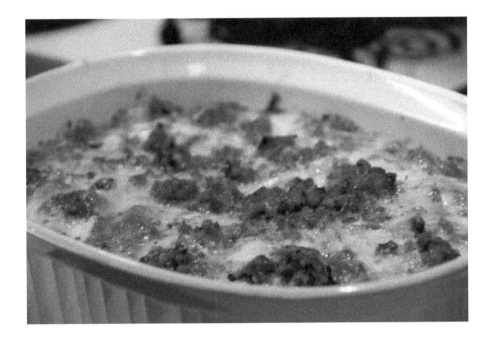

Zucchini Bread with Walnuts

Prep Time:
1 hour and 15 minutes
Serve: 16

Ingredients:

- 3 large organic eggs, beaten
- ½ cup of extra-virgin olive oil
- 1 cup of zucchini, finely grated
- ½ cup of walnuts, chopped
- 1 teaspoon of pure vanilla extract
- 2 ½ cups of almond flour
- ½ cup of erythritol or other keto-friendly sweeteners
- ½ teaspoon of fine sea salt
- 1 teaspoon of baking soda or baking powder
- ¼ teaspoon of grated ginger
- 1 teaspoon of cinnamon

Directions:

1.In a large bowl, add all the ingredients and gently stir until well blended.

2.Grease a 7-inch pan that fits inside your Instant Pot with nonstick cooking spray.

3.Add the bread batter to the pan and cover with aluminum foil.

4.Add 1 cup of water and place a trivet inside your Instant Pot. Place the pan on top of the trivet.

5.Lock the lid and cook at high pressure for 55 minutes. When the cooking is done, naturally release the pressure for 10 minutes. Carefully remove the lid. Unfold the aluminum foil and allow it to cool.

Nutrition: Calories: 200, Fat: 19g, Net Carb: 3g, Protein: 6g

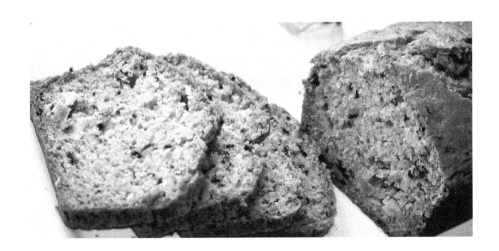

Breakfast Chicken and Egg

Prep Time:
30 minutes
Serve: 6

Ingredients:

- 1 pound of boneless, skinless chicken breasts
- 6 large organic eggs
- 2 tablespoons of extra-virgin olive oil
- 1 large onion, finely chopped
- 1 cup of water
- ½ cup of cauliflower rice
- 2 tablespoons of fresh parsley, finely chopped
- 1 teaspoon of fine sea salt
- 1 teaspoon of freshly cracked black pepper

Directions:

1.Press the "Sauté" function on your Instant Pot and add the olive oil. Once hot, add the onions and cook until fragrant, stirring occasionally. Remove and set aside.

2.Add the chicken and cook for 4 minutes per side or until brown.

3.Pour in 1 cup of water and lock the lid. Cook at high pressure for 15 minutes.

4.When the cooking is done, naturally release the pressure and remove the lid.

5.Transfer the chicken to a cutting board and shred using two forks.

6.In a large bowl, add the shredded chicken, eggs, onions, cauliflower rice, fresh parsley, salt, and black pepper. Stir until well combined.

7.Grease an oven-proof dish that fits inside your Instant Pot. Add the egg mixture and cover with foil.

8.Place a trivet inside your Instant Pot and place the dish on top. Lock the lid and cook at high pressure for another 8 minutes.

9.When the cooking is done, naturally release the pressure and remove the lid. Serve and enjoy!

Nutrition: Calories: 275, Fat: 13g, Net Carb: 2g, Protein: 35g

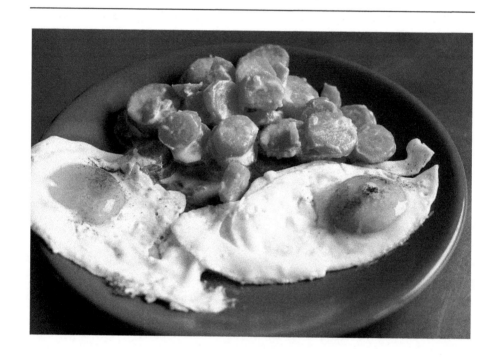

Eggs en Cocotte

Prep Time:
20 minutes
Serve: 3

Ingredients:

- 3 tablespoons of unsalted butter
- 3 tablespoons of heavy whipping cream
- 3 large organic eggs
- 1 tablespoon of fresh chives, chopped
- ½ teaspoon of fine sea salt
- ½ teaspoon of freshly cracked black pepper
- 1 cup of water

Directions:

1.Grease 3 ramekins with unsalted butter and add 1 tablespoon of heavy whipping cream into each one.

2.Crack an egg into each rameki
and sprinkle with fresh chives, salt, and black pepper.

3.Add 1 cup of water and a trivet inside your Instant Pot. Place the ramekins on top of the trivet and cover with aluminum foil. Lock the lid and cook at low pressure for 2 minutes.

4.When the timer beeps, naturally release the pressure and carefully remove the lid.

Nutrition: Calories: 420, Fat: 44.5g, Net Carbs: 0.8g, Protein: 6.2g

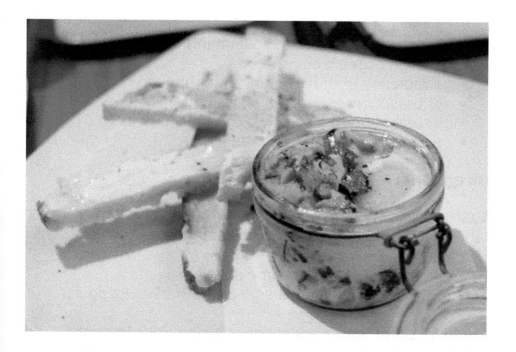

Breakfast Chocolate Zucchini Muffins

Prep Time:
40 minutes
Serve: Around 24 muffin bites

Ingredients:

- 2 large organic eggs
- ½ cup of coconut oil, melted
- 2 teaspoons of pure vanilla extract
- 1 tablespoon of unsalted butter
- 3 tablespoons of unsweetened cocoa powder
- 1 cup of almond flour
- ½ teaspoon of baking soda or baking powder
- 1 cup of evaporated cane juice
- 1 cup of water
- ½ teaspoon of ground cinnamon
- 1 cup of finely grated zucchini
- 1/3 cup of mini chocolate chips
- A small pinch of fine sea salt

Directions:

1. In a large bowl, add all the ingredients one by one and gently stir until well blended.

2. Fill silicone muffin cups with the batter.

3. Add 1 cup of water and a trivet inside your Instant Pot. Layer the muffins on top of the trivet. Cover with aluminum foil.

4.Lock the lid and cook at high pressure for 8 minutes. When the cooking is done, naturally release the pressure and remove the lid.

5.Remove the muffins and check if done using toothpicks.

Nutrition: Calories: 71, Fat: 6.8g, Net Carbs: 1.8g, Protein: 1g

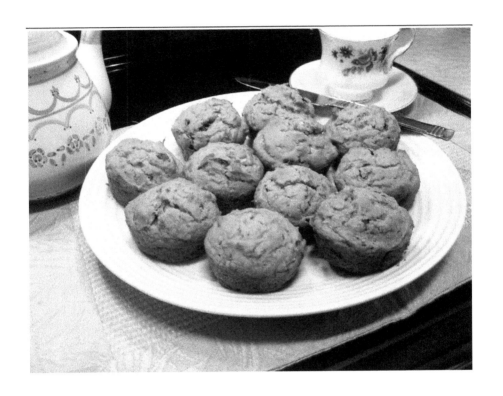

Cauliflower Oatmeal

Prep Time:
15 minutes
Serve: 1

Ingredients:

- 1 cup of fine cauliflower rice
- ½ cup of coconut cream
- ½ teaspoon of organic ground cinnamon
- ¼ teaspoon of granulated erythritol
- ½ tablespoon of peanut butter
- A small pinch of fine sea salt

Directions:

1.Add all the ingredients except for the peanut butter and stir until well combined.

2.Lock the lid and cook at high pressure for 2 minutes.

3.When the cooking is done, naturally release the pressure and remove the lid. Transfer to bowls and top with peanut butter.

Nutrition: Calories: 140, Fat: 7g, Net Carbs: 8g, Protein: 7g

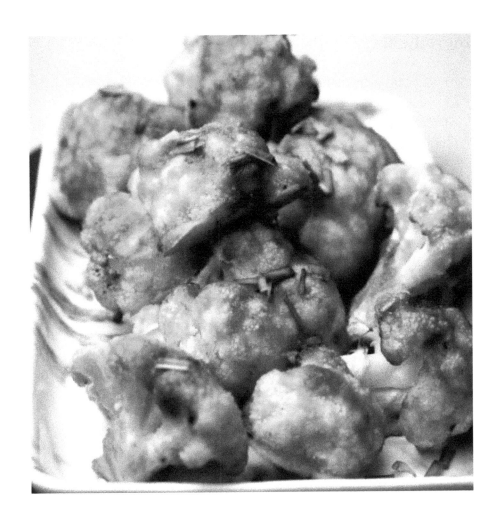

Chocolate Cauliflower Rice Pudding

Prep Time:
16 minutes
Serve: 2

Ingredients:

- 2 cups of fine cauliflower rice
- 1 cup of heavy whipping cream
- 1/3 cup of granulated erythritol or other keto-friendly sweeteners
- 1 to 2 egg whites
- 1 teaspoon of pure vanilla extract
- 3 tablespoons of unsweetened cocoa powder
- A small pinch of fine sea salt

Directions:

1.Add all the ingredients and stir until well combined.

2.Lock the lid and cook at high pressure for 2 minutes. When the cooking is done, naturally release the pressure and carefully remove the lid.

Nutrition: Calories: 313, Fat: 27.7g, Net Carbs: 5g, Protein: 10g

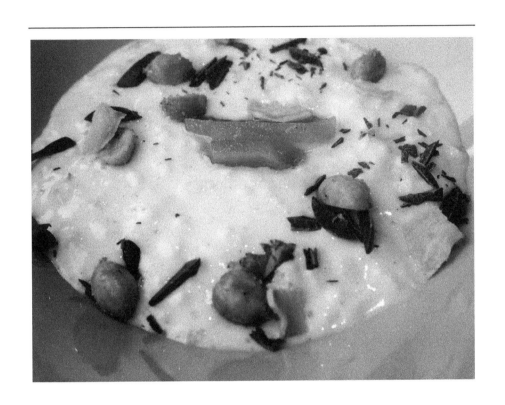

Mushroom and Cauliflower Risotto

Prep Time:
25 minutes
Serve: 4

Ingredients:

- 1 medium cauliflower head, cut into florets
- 1 pound of shiitake mushrooms, sliced
- 3 medium garlic cloves, peeled and minced
- 2 tablespoons of coconut aminos
- 1 cup of homemade low-sodium chicken stock
- 1 cup of full-fat coconut milk
- 1 tablespoon of coconut oil, melted
- 1 small onion, finely chopped
- 2 tablespoons of almond flour
- ¼ cup of nutritional yeast

Directions:

1.Press the "Sauté" function on your Instant Pot and add the coconut oil.

2.Once hot, add the onions, mushrooms, and garlic. Sauté for 5 minutes or until softened, stirring occasionally.

3.Add the remaining ingredients except for the almond flour. Lock the lid and cook at high pressure for 2 minutes.

4.When the cooking is done, naturally release the pressure and remove the lid.

5.Sprinkle the almond flour over the risotto and stir to thicken.

Nutrition: Calories: 230, Fat: 18.5g, Net Carbs: 8g, Protein: 7.5g

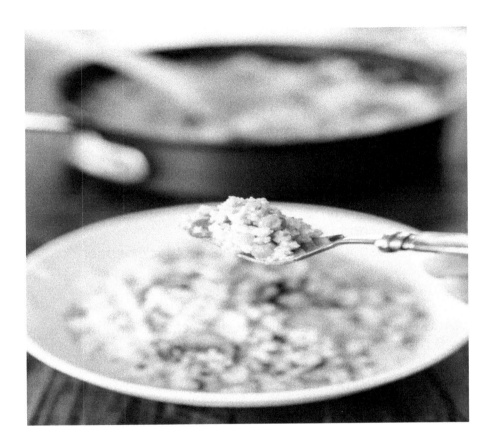

Coconut and Lime Cauliflower Rice

Prep Time:
15 minutes
Serve: 4

Ingredients:

- 1 large cauliflower, chopped
- 2 tablespoons of extra-virgin olive oil
- 1 large yellow onion, finely chopped
- 3 medium garlic cloves, peeled and minced
- 1 (15-ounce can of full-fat coconut milk
- 1 medium lime, zest, and juice
- ½ teaspoon of fine sea salt
- ¼ teaspoon of freshly cracked black pepper

Directions:

1.Add the cauliflowers to a food processor and pulse until they resemble rice-like consistency.

2.Press the "Sauté" function on your Instant Pot and add the olive oil. Once hot, add the onions and garlic. Sauté for 2 to 3 minutes or until fragrant, stirring occasionally.

3.Add the remaining ingredients and lock the lid. Cook at high pressure for 3 minutes.

4.When the cooking is done, quickly release the pressure and remove the lid.

Nutrition: Calories: 160, Fat: 11g, Net Carbs: 6g, Protein: 5g

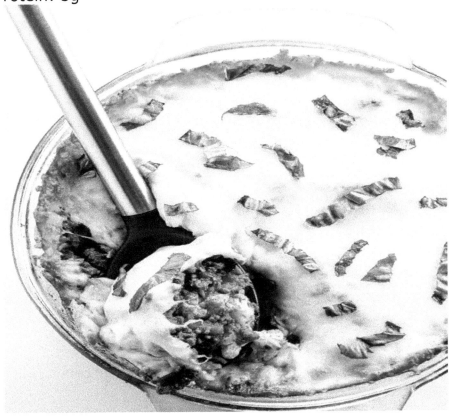

Eggs with Avocados and Feta Cheese

Prep Time:
10 minutes
Serve: 2

Ingredients:

- 4 large organic eggs
- 1 large avocado, peeled and cut into 12 slices
- 2 tablespoons of crumbled feta cheese
- 1 tablespoon of fresh parsley, finely chopped
- ½ teaspoon of fine sea salt
- ½ teaspoon of freshly cracked black pepper
- Grease 2 gratin dishes with nonstick cooking spray.

Directions:

1.Arrange 6 avocado slices into each gratin dish. Crack 2 eggs into each dish.

2.Sprinkle with crumbled feta cheese, fresh parsley, salt, and black pepper.

3.Wrap with aluminum foil.

4.Add 1 cup of water and a trivet inside your Instant Pot. Place the gratin dish on top of the trivet.

5.Lock the lid and cook at high pressure for 4 minutes. When the cooking is done, quick release or naturally release the pressure. Carefully remove the lid and check if the eggs are done.

Nutrition: Calories: 362, Fat: 30g, Net Carb: 4g, Protein: 16g

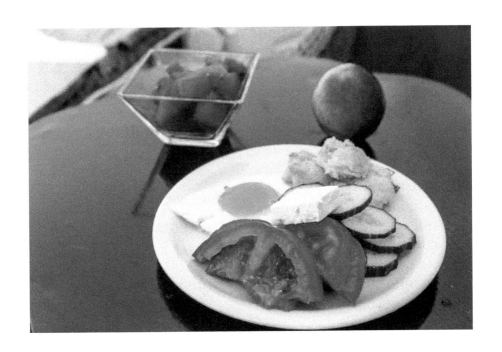

Giant Keto Pancake

Prep Time:
50 minutes
Serve: 6

Ingredients:

- 2 cups of almond flour or coconut flour
- 2 teaspoons of baking powder
- 2 tablespoons of granulated erythritol or another keto-friendly sweetener
- 2 large organic eggs
- 1 ½ cup of unsweetened almond milk or coconut milk

Directions:

1.In a large bowl, add all the ingredients and stir until well combined.

2.Grease a springform pan with nonstick cooking spray and add the pancake batter.

3.Add 1 cup of water and a trivet inside your Instant Pot. Place the springform pan on top of the trivet.

4.Lock the lid and cook at low pressure for 45 minutes. When the cooking is done, remove the lid and allow the pancake to cool.

Nutrition: Calories: 280, Fat: 24g, Net Carbs: 1g, Protein: 9g

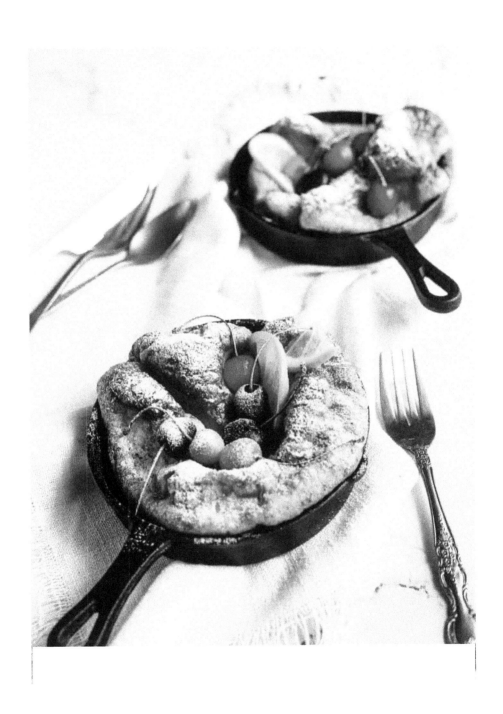

Breakfast Burrito Casserole

Prep Time:
25 minutes
Serve: 6

Ingredients:

- 4 large organic eggs
- 1 cup of cheddar cheese, cubed
- ¼ cup of white or yellow onion, finely chopped
- 1 medium jalapeno, finely chopped
- 1 cup of cooked ham, cut into cubes
- ½ teaspoon of fine sea salt
- ½ teaspoon of freshly cracked black pepper
- ½ teaspoon of chili powder
- Lettuce leaves

Directions:

1.In a large bowl, add all the ingredients and stir until well combined.

2.Grease a springform pan or a round metal bowl with nonstick cooking spray.

3.Add the egg mixture.

4.Add 1 cup of water and a trivet inside your Instant Pot. Place the pan on top of the trivet and cover with aluminum foil.

5.Lock the lid and cook at high pressure for 12 minutes. When the cooking is done, naturally release the pressure and remove the lid.

6.Remove the pan and spoon the egg mixture onto lettuce leaves. Top with salsa and avocado slices.

Nutrition: Calories: 165, Fat: 11.5g, Net Carbs: 1.5g, Protein: 13g

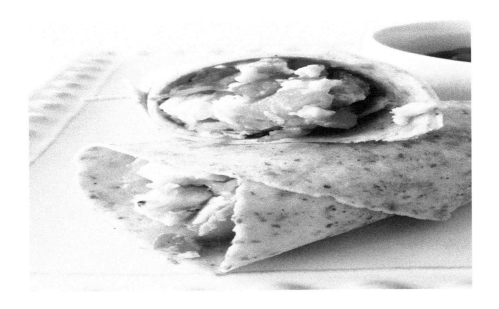

Breakfast Ratatouille

Prep Time:
30 minutes
Serve: 6

Ingredients:

- 12 large organic eggs
- ¼ cup of extra-virgin olive oil
- 1 medium yellow onion, finely chopped
- 6 medium garlic cloves, peeled and finely minced
- 1 (28-ounce can of plum tomatoes, drained
- 1 medium eggplant, chopped
- 1 zucchini, sliced
- 1 medium yellow bell pepper, seeded and chopped
- 1 tablespoon of capers, chopped
- 1 tablespoon of red wine vinegar
- 2 teaspoons of fresh thyme, finely chopped
- 1 teaspoon of fresh oregano, finely chopped
- 3 tablespoons of fresh basil, finely chopped
- 3 tablespoons of fresh parsley, finely chopped

Directions:

1.Press the "Sauté" function on your Instant Pot and add olive oil and onions.

2.Sauté for 4 minutes or until slightly softened, stirring occasionally.

3.Add the garlic and herbs. Sauté until fragrant, stirring occasionally.

4.Add the tomatoes, eggplant, bell peppers, and zucchini. Stir until well combined.

5.Lock the lid and cook at high pressure for 5 minutes. When the cooking is done, quickly release the pressure and remove the lid.

6.Stir in the capers and red wine vinegar.

7.In a small skillet over medium-high heat, add the vegetables. Make small cavities and crack eggs into the cavity. Cover and allow the eggs to cook through.

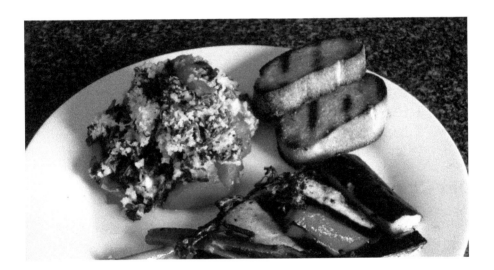

Spanish Chorizo and Cauliflower Hash

Prep Time:
20 minutes
Serve: 4

Ingredients:

- 1 pound of cauliflower florets, cut into florets
- 1 tablespoon of extra-virgin olive oil
- 1 medium sweet potato, cut into bite-sized pieces
- 1 pound of chorizo sausage, crumbled
- 1 large onion, finely chopped
- 2 medium garlic cloves, peeled and minced
- 3 tablespoons of fresh rosemary, finely chopped
- 3 tablespoons of fresh basil, finely chopped
- 1 teaspoon of fine sea salt
- 1 teaspoon of freshly cracked black pepper
- ½ cup of homemade low-sodium vegetable stock

Directions:

1.Press the "Sauté" function on your Instant Pot and add the olive oil. Once hot, add the onions and garlic. Sauté for 2 minutes or until softened, stirring occasionally.

2.Add the sweet potato pieces, chorizo sausage, and cauliflower. Sauté for 3 minutes, stirring occasionally.

3.Add the remaining ingredients and stir until well combined.

4.Pour in the vegetable stock and lock the lid. Cook at high pressure for 10 minutes. When the cooking is done, naturally release the pressure and remove the lid. Serve and enjoy!

Nutrition: Calories: 550, Fat: 35g, Net Carbs: 12g, Protein: 23g

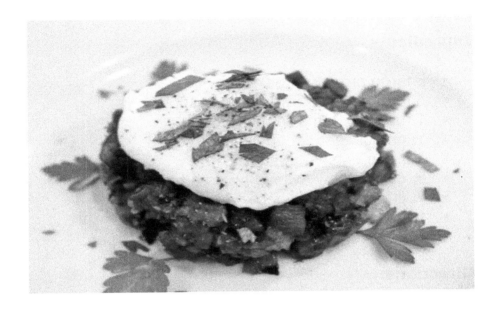

BLT Egg Casserole

Prep Time:
 30 minutes
Serve: 4

Ingredients:

- 6 large organic eggs
- 6 medium slices of bacon, chopped
- 1 medium Roma tomato, sliced
- ½ cup of cheddar cheese, shredded
- 2 green onions, thinly sliced
- ½ cup of heavy whipping cream
- ½ cup of fresh spinach
- 1 teaspoon of fine sea salt
- 1 teaspoon of freshly cracked black pepper

Directions:

1.In a large bowl, add all the ingredients and stir until well combined.

2.Grease a large springform pan with nonstick cooking spray and add the egg mixture.

3.Add 1 cup of water and place a trivet inside your Instant Pot. Place the springform pan on top of the trivet and cover with aluminum foil.

4.Lock the lid and cook at high pressure for 13 minutes.

5.When the cooking is done, naturally release the pressure for 10 minutes, then quickly release the remaining pressure. Remove the lid.

Nutrition: Calories: 360, Fat: 29g, Net Carbs: 2g, Protein: 23g

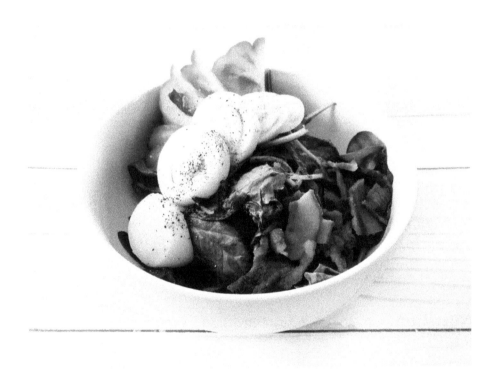

Coconut Oatmeal

Prep Time:
20 minutes
Serve: 4

Ingredients:

- 2 cups almond milk
- 1 cup coconut; shredded
- 2 tsp. vanilla extract
- 2 tsp. stevia

Directions:

1.In a pan that fits your air fryer, mix all the ingredients, stir well, introduce the pan in the machine and cook at 360°F for 15 minutes

2.Divide into bowls and serve for breakfast.

Nutrition: Calories: 201; Fat: 13g; Fiber: 2g; Carbs: 4g; Protein: 7g

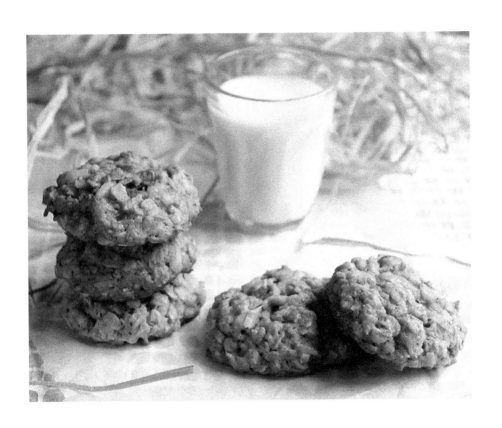

Cheesy Tomatoes

Prep Time:
20 minutes
Serve: 4

Ingredients:

- 1 lb. cherry tomatoes; halved
- 1 cup mozzarella; shredded
- 1 tsp. basil; chopped.
- Cooking spray
- Salt and black pepper to taste.

Directions:

1.Grease the tomatoes with the cooking spray, season with salt and pepper, sprinkle the mozzarella on top, place them all in your air fryer's basket, cook at 330°F for 15 minutes

2.Divide into bowls, sprinkle the basil on top, and serve.

Nutrition: Calories: 140; Fat: 7g; Fiber: 3g; Carbs: 4g; Protein: 5g

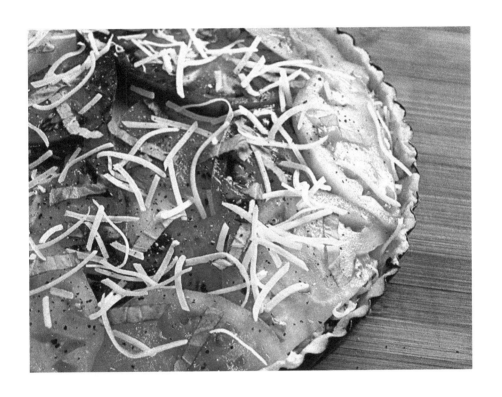

Banana Nut Cake

Prep Time:
35 minutes
Serve: 6

Ingredients:

- 1 cup blanched finely ground almond flour
- 2 large eggs.
- ¼ cup unsalted butter; melted.
- ¼ cup full-fat sour cream.
- ¼ cup chopped walnuts
- ½ cup powdered erythritol
- 2 tbsp. ground golden flaxseed.
- 2 ½ tsp. banana extract.
- 1 tsp. Vanilla extract.
- 2 tsp. baking powder.
- ½ tsp. Ground cinnamon.

Directions:

1.Take a large bowl, mix almond flour, erythritol, flaxseed, baking powder, and cinnamon. Stir in butter, banana extract, vanilla extract, and sour cream

2.Add eggs to the mixture and gently stir until fully combined. Stir in the walnuts

3.Pour into a 6-inch nonstick cake pan and place into the air fryer basket. Adjust the temperature to 300 Degrees F and set the timer for 25 minutes

4.Cake will be golden, and a toothpick inserted in the center will come out clean when fully cooked. Allow to fully cool to avoid crumbling.

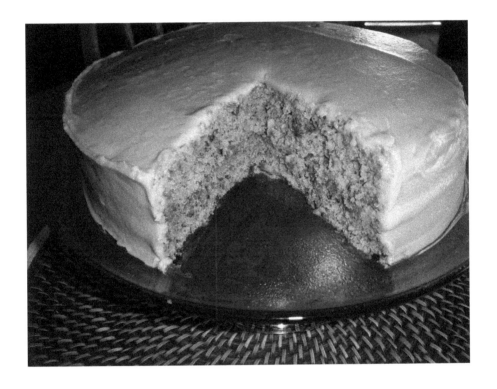

Nutrition: Calories: 263; Protein: 7.6g; Fiber: 3.1g; Fat: 23.6g; Carbs: 18.4g

Olives and Kale

Prep Time:
25 minutes
Serve: 4

Ingredients:

- 4 eggs; whisked
- 1 cup kale; chopped.
- ½ cup black olives, pitted and sliced
- 2 tbsp. cheddar; grated Cooking spray
- A pinch of salt and black pepper

Directions:

1. Take a bowl and mix the eggs with the rest of the ingredients except the cooking spray and whisk well.

2. Now, take a pan that fits in your air fryer and grease it with the cooking spray, pour the olives mixture inside, spread

3. Put the pan into the machine and cook at 360°F for 20 minutes. Serve for breakfast hot.

Nutrition: Calories: 220; Fat: 13g; Fiber: 4g; Carbs: 6g; Protein: 12g

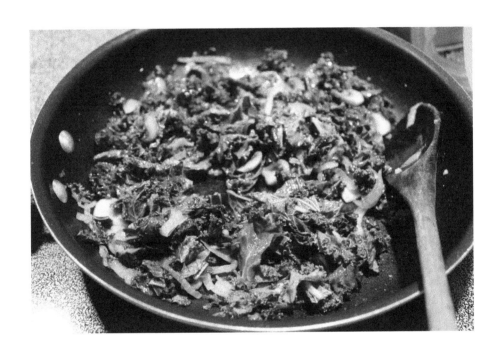

Cheesy Turkey

Prep Time:
30 minutes
Serve: 4

Ingredients:

- 1 turkey breast, skinless, boneless; cut into strips and browned
- 2 cups almond milk
- 2 cups cheddar cheese; shredded
- 2 eggs; whisked
- 2 tsp. olive oil
- 1 tbsp. chives; chopped.
- Salt and black pepper to taste.

Directions:

1.Take a bowl and mix the eggs with milk, cheese, salt, pepper, and the chives and whisk well.

2.Preheat the air fryer at 330°F, add the oil, heat it, add the turkey pieces and spread them well

3.Add the egg mixture, toss a bit, and cook for 25 minutes.

Nutrition: Calories: 244; Fat: 11g; Fiber: 4g; Carbs: 5g; Protein: 7g

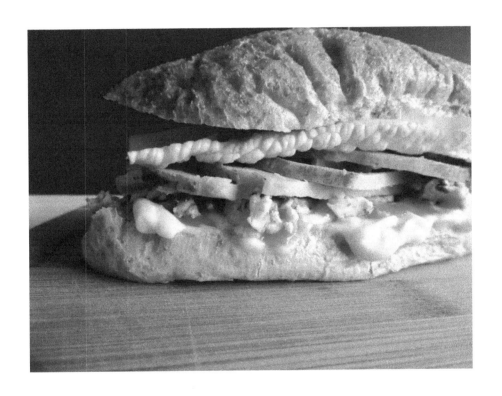

Mushrooms and Cheese Spread

Prep Time:
25 minutes
Serve: 4

Ingredients:

- ¼ cup mozzarella; shredded
- ½ cup coconut cream
- 1 cup white mushrooms
- A pinch of salt and black pepper
- Cooking spray

Directions:

1.Put the mushrooms in your air fryer's basket, grease with cooking spray, and cook at 370°F for 20 minutes.

2.Transfer to a blender, add the remaining ingredients, pulse well, divide into bowls and serve as a spread.

Nutrition: Calories: 202; Fat: 12g; Fiber: 2g; Carbs: 5g; Protein: 7g

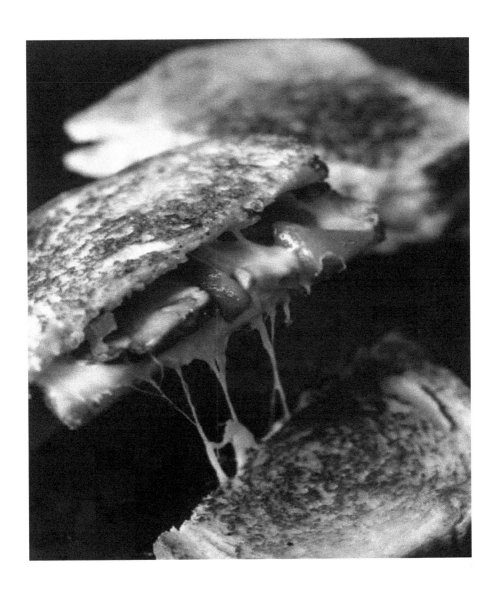

Cheesy Sausage Balls

Prep Time:
22 minutes
Serve: 16 balls

Ingredients:

- 1 lb. pork breakfast sausage
- 1 large egg.
- 1 oz. full-fat cream cheese; softened.
- ½ cup shredded Cheddar cheese

Directions:

1.Mix all ingredients in a large bowl. Form into sixteen (1-inch balls. Place the balls into the air fryer basket.

2.Adjust the temperature to 400 Degrees F and set the timer for 12 minutes. Shake the basket two or three times during cooking

3.Sausage balls will be browned on the outside and have an internal temperature of at least 145 Degrees F when completely cooked.

Nutrition: Calories: 424; Protein: 22.8g; Fiber: 0.0g; Fat: 32.2g; Carbs: 1.6g

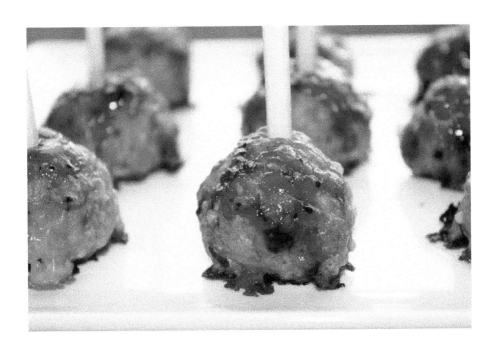

Blackberries Bowls

Prep Time:
20 minutes
Serve: 4

Ingredients:

- 1 ½ cups coconut milk
- ½ cup coconut; shredded
- ½ cup blackberries
- 2 tsp. stevia

Directions:

1.In your air fryer's pan, mix all the ingredients, stir, cover and cook at 360°F for 15 minutes.

Nutrition: Calories: 171; Fat: 4g; Fiber: 2g; Carbs: 3g; Protein: 5g

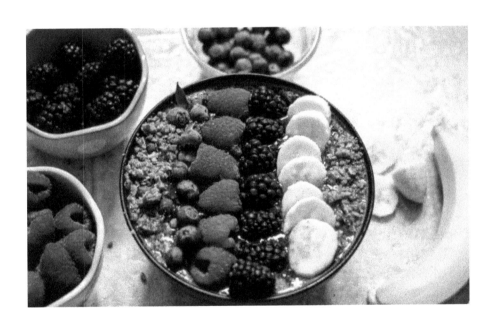

Cilantro Omelet

Prep Time:
25 minutes
Serve: 4

Ingredients:

- 6 eggs; whisked
- 1 cup mozzarella; shredded
- 1 cup cilantro; chopped.
- Cooking spray
- Salt and black pepper to taste.

Directions:

1.Take a bowl and mix all the ingredients except the cooking spray and whisk well.

2.Grease a pan that fits your air fryer with the cooking spray, pour the eggs mix, spread, put the pan into the machine, and cook at 350°F for 20 minutes

3.Divide the omelet between plates and serve for breakfast.

Nutrition: Calories: 270; Fat: 15g; Fiber: 3g; Carbs: 5g; Protein: 9g

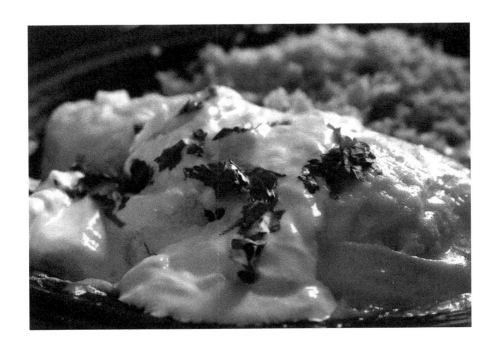

Tomatoes and Swiss Chard Bake

Prep Time:
20 minutes
Serve: 4

Ingredients:

- 4 eggs; whisked
- 3 oz. Swiss chard; chopped.
- 1 cup tomatoes; cubed
- 1 tsp. olive oil
- Salt and black pepper to taste.

Directions:

1.Take a bowl and mix the eggs with the rest of the ingredients except the oil and whisk well.

2.Grease a pan that fits the fryer with the oil, pour the swiss chard mix and cook at 359°F for 15 minutes.

Nutrition: Calories: 202; Fat: 14g; Fiber: 3g; Carbs: 5g; Protein: 12g

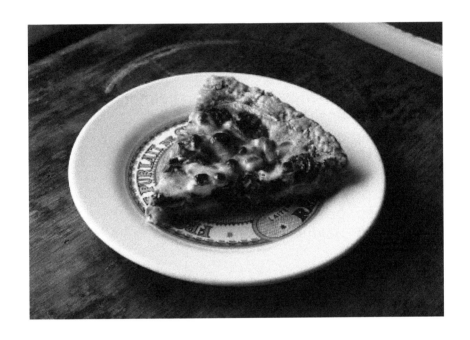

Pumpkin Spice Muffins

Prep Time:
25 minutes
Serve: 6

Ingredients:

- 2 large eggs.
- 1 cup blanched finely ground almond flour.
- ¼ cup unsalted butter; softened.
- ¼ cup pure pumpkin purée.
- ½ cup granular erythritol.
- ¼ tsp. Ground nutmeg.
- 1 tsp. vanilla extract.
- ½ tsp. ground cinnamon.
- ½ tsp. Baking powder.

Directions:

1.Take a large bowl, mix almond flour, erythritol, baking powder, butter, pumpkin purée, cinnamon, nutmeg, and vanilla. Gently stir in eggs.

2.Evenly pour the batter into six silicone muffin cups. Place muffin cups into the air fryer basket, working in batches if necessary.

3.Adjust the temperature to 300 Degrees F and set the timer for 15 minutes. When completely cooked, a toothpick inserted in the center will come out mostly clean. Serve warm.

Nutrition: Calories: 205; Protein: 6.3g; Fiber: 2.4g; Fat: 18.0g; Carbs: 17.4g

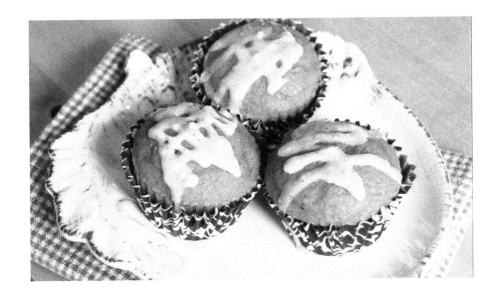

Strawberries Oatmeal

Prep Time:
20 minutes
Serve: 4

Ingredients:

- ½ cup coconut; shredded
- ¼ cup strawberries
- 2 cups coconut milk
- ¼ tsp. vanilla extract 2 tsp. stevia
- Cooking spray

Directions:

1.Grease the Air Fryer's pan with the cooking spray, add all the ingredients inside, and toss

2.Cook at 365°F for 15 minutes, divide into bowls and serve for breakfast.

Nutrition: Calories: 142; Fat: 7g; Fiber: 2g; Carbs: 3g; Protein: 5g

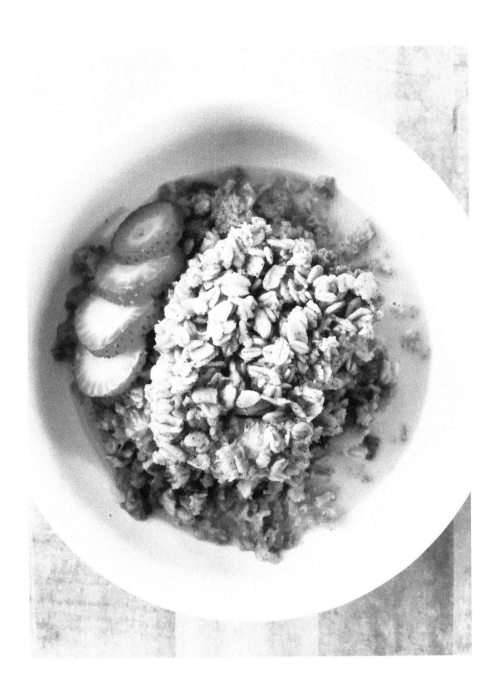

Tuna and Spring Onions Salad

Prep Time:
20 minutes
Serve: 4

Ingredients:

- 14 oz. canned tuna drained and flaked
- 2 spring onions; chopped.
- 1 cup arugula
- 1 tbsp. olive oil
- A pinch of salt and black pepper

Directions:

1.In a bowl, all the ingredients except the oil and the arugula and whisk.

2.Preheat the Air Fryer over 360°F, add the oil, and grease it. Pour the tuna mix, stir well and cook for 15 minutes

3.In a salad bowl, combine the arugula with the tuna mix, toss and serve.

Nutrition: Calories: 212; Fat: 8g; Fiber: 3g; Carbs: 5g; Protein: 8g

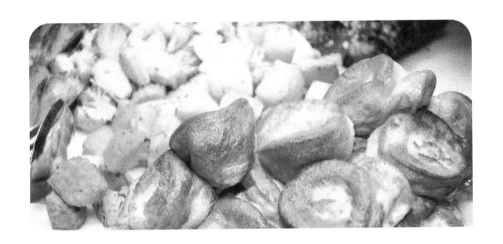

Scrambled Eggs

Prep Time:
 20 minutes
Serve: 2

Ingredients:

- 4 large eggs.
- ½ cup shredded sharp Cheddar cheese.
- 2 tbsp. unsalted butter; melted.

Directions:

1.Crack eggs into a 2-cup round baking dish and whisk. Place dish into the air fryer basket.

2.Adjust the temperature to 400 Degrees F and set the timer for 10 minutes

3.After 5 minutes, stir the eggs and add the butter and cheese. Let cook 3 more minutes and stir again

4.Allow eggs to finish cooking for an additional 2 minutes or remove if they are to your desired liking. Use a fork to fluff.

Nutrition: Calories: 359; Protein: 19.5g; Fiber: 0.0g; Fat: 27.6g; Carbs: 1.1g

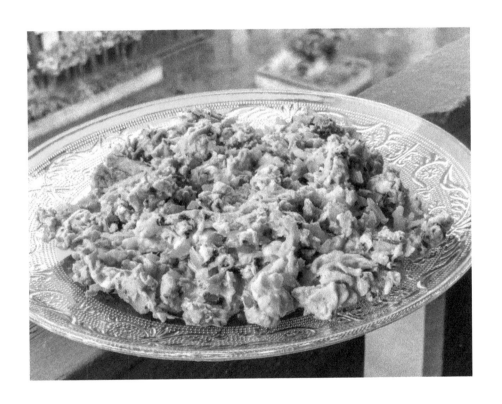

Herbed Eggs

Prep Time:
25 minutes
Serve: 4

Ingredients:

- ½ cup cheddar; shredded
- 10 eggs; whisked
- 2 tbsp. chives; chopped.
- 2 tbsp. basil; chopped.
- 2 tbsp. parsley; chopped. Cooking spray
- Salt and black pepper to taste.

Directions:

1.Take a bowl and mix the eggs with all the ingredients except the cheese and the cooking spray and whisk well

2.Preheat the air fryer at 350°F, grease it with the cooking spray, and pour the eggs mixture inside

3.Sprinkle the cheese on top and cook for 20 minutes. Divide everything between plates and serve.

Nutrition: Calories: 232; Fat: 12g; Fiber: 4g; Carbs: 5g; Protein: 7g

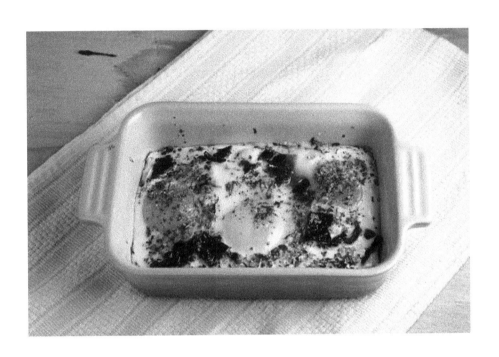

Cherry Tomatoes Omelet

Prep Time:
25 minutes
Serve: 4

Ingredients:

- 1 lb. cherry tomatoes; halved
- 4 eggs; whisked
- 1 tbsp. cheddar; grated
- 1 tbsp. parsley; chopped.
- Salt and black pepper to taste.
- Cooking spray

Directions:

1.Put the tomatoes in the air fryer's basket, cook at 360°F for 5 minutes and transfer them to the baking pan that fits the machine greased with cooking spray

2.Take a bowl, mix the eggs with the remaining ingredients, whisk, pour over the tomatoes, and cook at 360°F for 15 minutes.

Nutrition: Calories: 230; Fat: 14g; Fiber: 3g; Carbs: 5g; Protein: 11g

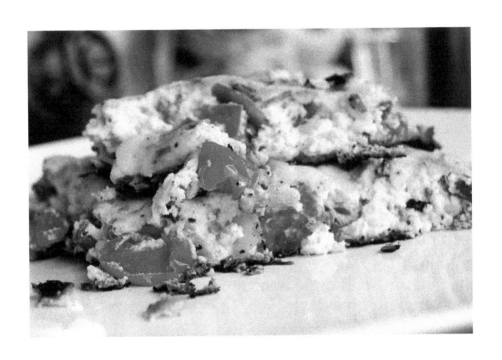

Basil Eggs

Prep Time:
25 minutes
Serve: 4

Ingredients:

- 1 cup mozzarella cheese; grated
- 6 eggs; whisked
- 2 tbsp. basil; chopped.
- 2 tbsp. butter; melted
- 6 tsp. basil pesto
- A pinch of salt and black pepper

Directions:

1.Take a bowl and mix all the ingredients except the butter and whisk them well.

2.Preheat your Air Fryer at 360°F, drizzle the butter on the bottom, spread the eggs mix, cook for 20 minutes and serve for breakfast

Nutrition: Calories: 207; Fat: 14g; Fiber: 3g; Carbs: 4g; Protein: 8g

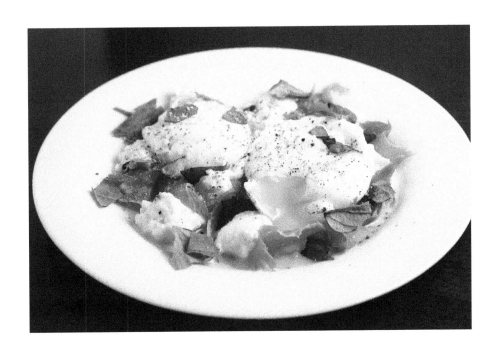

Zucchini and Artichokes Mix

Prep Time:
25 minutes
Serve: 4

Ingredients:

- 8 oz. canned artichokes, drained and chopped.
- 2 tomatoes; cut into quarters
- 4 eggs; whisked
- 4 spring onions; chopped.
- 2 zucchinis; sliced
- Cooking spray
- Salt and black pepper to taste.

Directions:

1.Grease a pan with cooking spray and mix all the other ingredients inside.

2.Put the pan in the Air Fryer and cook at 350°F for 20 minutes. Divide between plates and serve

Nutrition: Calories: 210; Fat: 11g; Fiber: 3g; Carbs: 4g; Protein: 6g

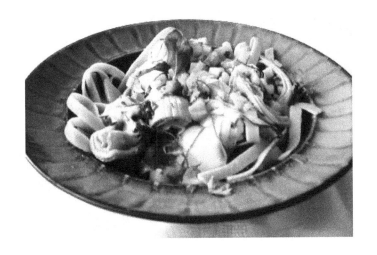

Paprika Eggs and Broccoli

Prep Time:
25 minutes
Serve: 4

Ingredients:

- 1 broccoli head, florets separated and roughly chopped.
- 4 oz. sour cream
- Cooking spray
- 2 eggs; whisked
- Salt and black pepper to taste.
- 1 tbsp. sweet paprika

Directions:

1.Grease a pan that fits your air fryer with the cooking spray and mix all the ingredients inside.

2.Put the pan in the Air Fryer and cook at 360°F for 20 minutes. Divide between plates and serve

Nutrition: Calories: 220; Fat: 14g; Fiber: 2g; Carbs: 3g; Protein: 2g

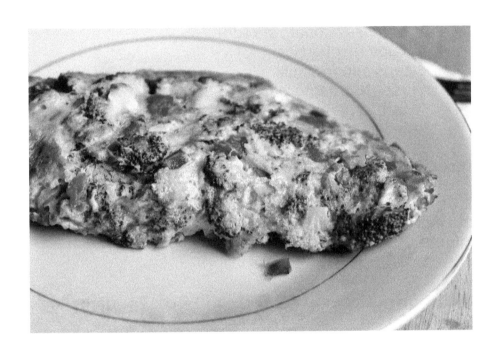

Raspberries Oatmeal

Prep Time:
20 minutes
Serve: 4

Ingredients:

- 1 ½ cups coconut; shredded
- ½ cups raspberries
- 2 cups almond milk
- ¼ tsp. Nutmeg ground 2 tsp. stevia
- ½ tsp. cinnamon powder
- Cooking spray

Directions:

1.Grease the air fryer's pan with cooking spray, mix all the ingredients inside, cover and cook at 360°F for 15 minutes.

Nutrition: Calories: 172; Fat: 5g; Fiber: 2g; Carbs: 4g; Protein: 6g

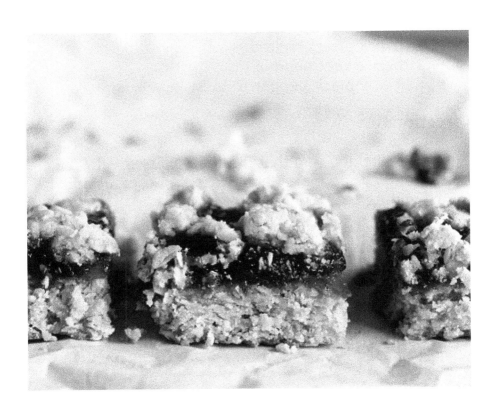

Zucchini Spread

Prep Time:
20 minutes
Serve: 4

Ingredients:

- 4 zucchinis; roughly chopped.
- 1 tbsp. butter; melted
- 1 tbsp. sweet paprika
- Salt and black pepper to taste.

Directions:

1.Grease a baking pan that fits the Air Fryer with the butter, add all the ingredients, toss and cook at 360°F for 15 minutes.

2.Transfer to a blender, pulse well, divide into bowls and serve for breakfast.

Nutrition: Calories: 240; Fat: 14g; Fiber: 2g; Carbs: 5g; Protein: 11g

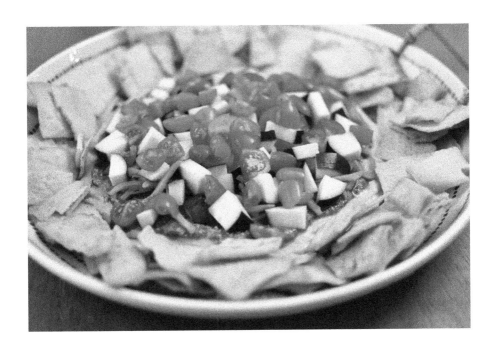

Breakfast Kale Frittata

Prep Time:
10 minutes

Cook Time:
30 minutes

Serve: 4

Ingredients:

- 6 kale stalks, chopped
- 1 small sweet onion, chopped
- 1 small broccoli head, florets separated
- 2 garlic cloves, minced
- Salt and black pepper to the taste
- 4 eggs
- 1 tablespoon olive oil

Directions:

1.Heat a pan with the oil over medium-high heat, add the onion, stir and cook for 4-5 minutes.

2.Add the garlic, broccoli, and kale, toss, and cook for 5 minutes more.

3.Add the eggs, salt, and pepper and mix. Place in the oven and bake at 380 degrees F for 20 minutes. Slice and serve for breakfast.

Nutrition: calories 214, fat 7, fiber 2, carbs 12, protein 8 13.

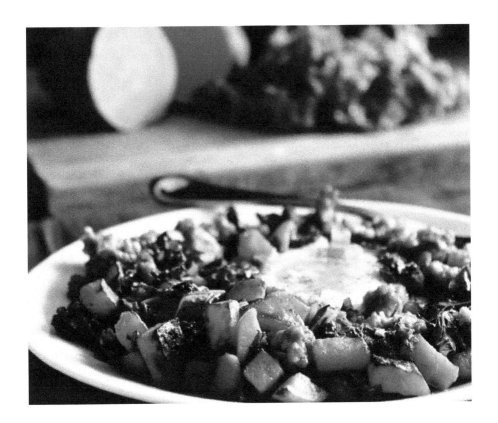

Cranberry Granola Bars

Prep Time:
2 h
Serve: 4

Ingredients:

- 2 cups walnuts, toasted
- 1 cup dates, pitted
- 3 tablespoons water
- ¾ cup cranberries, dried, no added sugar
- 2 cups desiccated coconut, unsweetened

Directions:

1.In your food processor, mix dates with coconut, cranberries, water, and walnuts.

2.Pulse well, then spread the mix into a lined baking dish. Press well into the dish and keep in the fridge for 2 hours, then cut into bars and serve.

Nutrition: calories 476, fat 40, fiber 9, carbs 33, protein 6

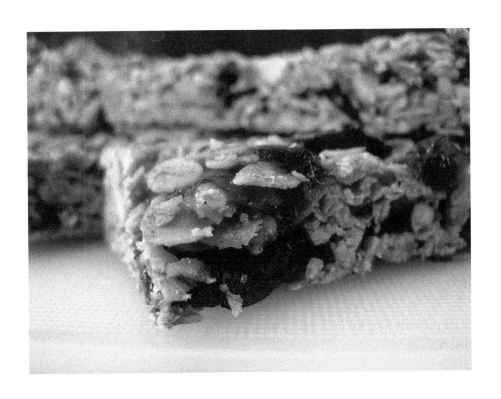

Spinach and Berry Smoothie

Prep Time:
10 min
Serve: 2

Ingredients:

- 1 cup blackberries
- 1 avocado, pitted, peeled, and chopped
- 1 banana, peeled and roughly chopped
- 1 cup baby spinach
- 1 tablespoon hemp seeds
- 1 cup water
- ½ cup almond milk, unsweetened

Directions:

1.In your blender, mix the berries with the avocado, banana, spinach, hemp seeds, water, and almond milk. Pulse well, divide into 2 glasses, and serve for breakfast.

Nutrition: calories 160, fat 3, fiber 4, carbs 6, protein 3 15.

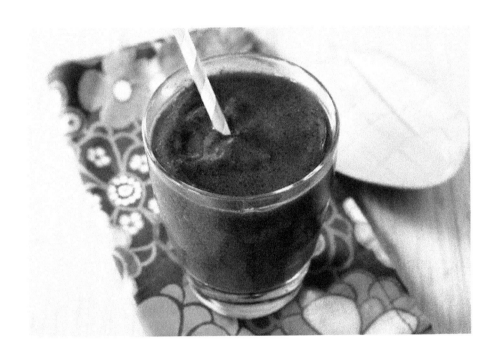

Zucchini Breakfast Salad

Prep Time:
10 min
Serve: 4

Ingredients:

- 2 zucchinis, spiralized
- 1 cup beets, baked, peeled, and grated
- ½ bunch kale, chopped
- 2 tablespoons olive oil

For the tahini sauce:
- 1 tablespoon maple syrup
- Juice of 1 lime
- ¼ inch fresh ginger, grated
- 1/3 cup sesame seed paste

Directions:

1.In a salad bowl, mix the zucchinis with the beets, kale, and oil.

2.In another small bowl, whisk the maple syrup with lime juice, ginger, and sesame paste. Pour the dressing over the salad, toss and serve it for breakfast.

Nutrition: calories 183, fat 3, fiber 2, carbs 7, protein 9 16.

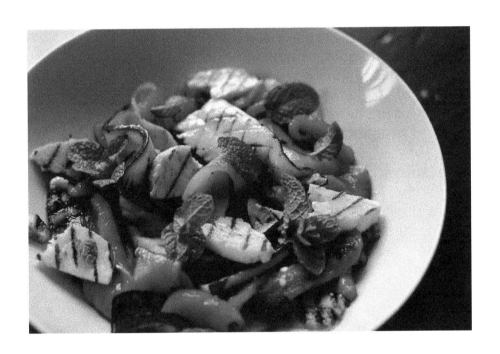

Quinoa and Spinach Breakfast Salad

Prep Time:
10 min
Cook Time:
0 min
Serve: 2

- 16 ounces quinoa, cooked
- 1 handful raisins
- 1 handful baby spinach leaves
- 1 tablespoon maple syrup
- ½ tablespoon lemon juice
- 4 tablespoons olive oil
- 1 teaspoon ground cumin
- A pinch of sea salt and black pepper
- ½ teaspoon chili flakes

Directions:

1.In a bowl, mix the quinoa with spinach, raisins, cumin, salt, pepper, and toss.

2.Add the maple syrup, lemon juice, oil, and chili flakes and toss, then serve for breakfast.

Nutrition: calories 170, fat 3, fiber 6, carbs 8, protein 5 17.

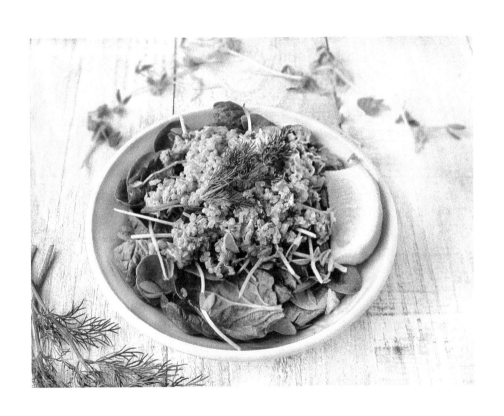

Carrots Breakfast Mix

Prep Time:
10 min
Cook Time:
0 min
Serve: 4

Ingredients:

- 1½ tablespoon maple syrup
- 1 teaspoon olive oil
- 1 tablespoon chopped walnuts
- 1 onion, chopped
- 4 cups shredded carrots
- 1 tablespoon curry powder
- ¼ teaspoon ground turmeric
- Black pepper to the taste
- 2 tablespoons sesame seed paste
- ¼ cup lemon juice
- ½ cup chopped parsley

Directions:

1.In a salad bowl, mix the onion with the carrots, turmeric, curry powder, black pepper, lemon juice, and parsley.

2.Add the maple syrup, oil, walnuts, and sesame seed paste. toss well and serve for breakfast.

Nutrition: calories 150, fat 3, fiber 2, carbs 6, protein 8 18.

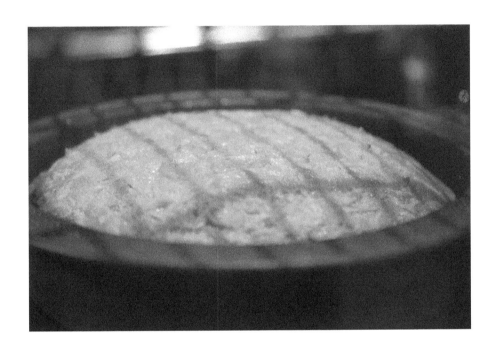

Italian Breakfast Salad

Prep Time:
10 min
Cook Time:
0 min
Serve: 4

Ingredients:

- 1 handful kalamata olives, pitted and sliced
- 1 cup cherry tomatoes, halved
- 1½ cucumbers, sliced
- 1 red onion, chopped
- 2 tablespoons chopped oregano
- 1 tablespoon chopped mint

For the salad dressing:
- 2 tablespoons balsamic vinegar
- ¼ cup olive oil
- 1 garlic clove, minced
- 2 teaspoons dried Italian herbs
- A pinch of salt and black pepper

Directions:

1.In a salad bowl, toss together the olives with the tomatoes, cucumbers, onion, mint, and oregano.

2.In a smaller bowl, whisk the vinegar with the oil, garlic, Italian herbs, salt, and pepper. Pour the dressing over the salad, toss and serve for breakfast.

Nutrition: calories 191, fat 10, fiber 3, carbs 13, protein 1

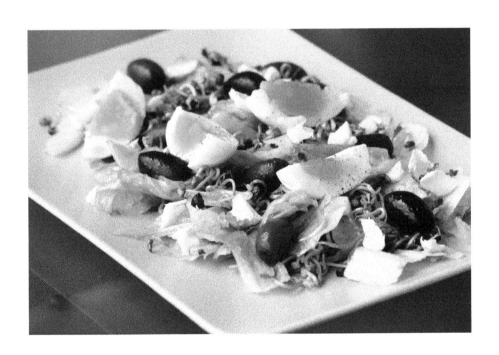

Zucchini and Sprout Breakfast Mix

Prep Time:
10 min
Cook Time:
0 min
Serve: 4

Ingredients:

- 2 zucchinis, spiralized
- 2 cups bean sprouts
- 4 green onions, chopped
- 1 red bell pepper, chopped
- Juice of 1 lime
- 1 tablespoon olive oil
- ½ cup chopped cilantro
- ¾ cup almonds chopped
- A pinch of salt and black pepper

Directions:

1.In a salad bowl, toss together the zucchinis with the bean sprouts, green onions, bell pepper, cilantro, almonds, salt, pepper, lime juice, and oil. Serve for breakfast.

Nutrition: calories 140, fat 4, fiber 2, carbs 7, protein 8 20.

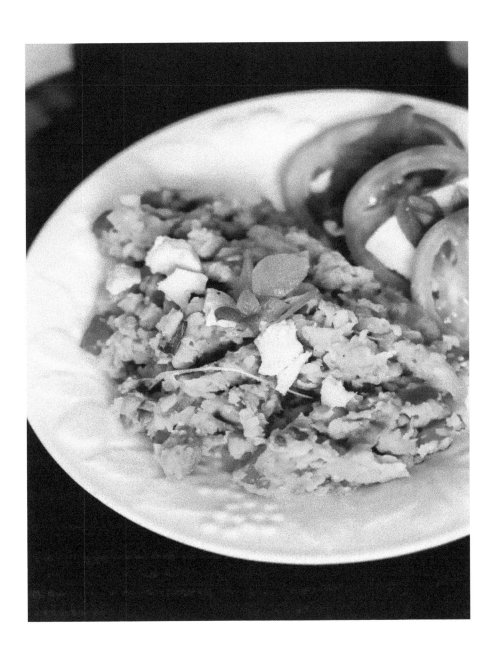

Breakfast Corn Salad

Prep Time:
10 min
Cook Time:
0 min
Serve: 4

Ingredients:

- 2 avocados, pitted, peeled, and cubed
- 1-pint mixed cherry tomatoes halved
- 2 cups fresh corn kernels
- 1 red onion, chopped

For the salad dressing:
- 2 tablespoons olive oil
- 1 tablespoon lime juice
- ½ teaspoon grated lime zest
- A pinch of salt and black pepper
- ¼ cup chopped cilantro

Directions:

1.In a salad bowl, mix the avocados with tomatoes, corn, and onion.

2.Add the oil, lime juice, lime zest, salt, pepper, and cilantro, toss and serve for breakfast.

Nutrition: calories 140, fat 3, fiber 2, carbs 6, protein 9 21.

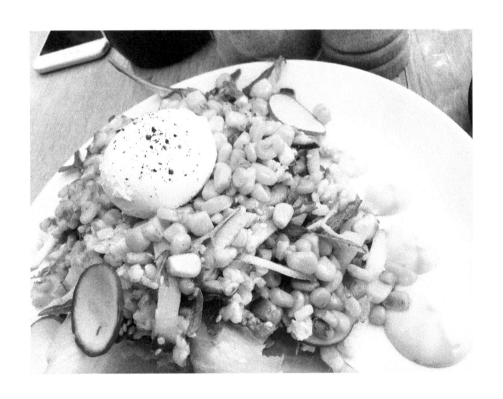

Simple Basil Tomato Mix

Prep Time:
10 min
Cook Time:
0 min
Serve: 6

Ingredients:

- ½ cup extra-virgin olive oil
- 1 cucumber, chopped
- 2 pints colored cherry tomatoes, halved Salt, and black pepper to the taste
- 1 red onion, chopped
- 3 tablespoons red vinegar
- 1 garlic clove, minced
- 1 bunch basil, roughly chopped

Directions:

1.In a salad bowl, toss together the cucumber with the tomatoes, onion, salt, pepper, oil, vinegar, basil, and garlic.

Nutrition: calories 100, fat 1, fiber 2, carbs 2, protein 6 22.

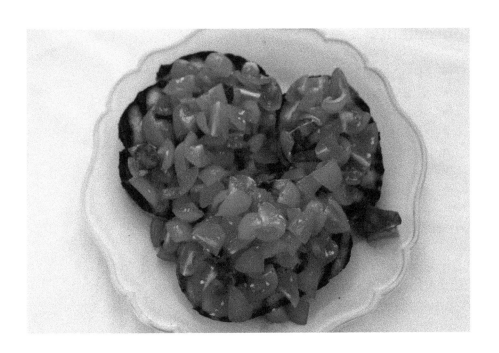

Cucumber and Avocado Salad

Prep Time:
10 min
Cook Time:
0 min
Serve: 4

Ingredients:

- 1 pound cucumbers, chopped
- 2 avocados, pitted and chopped
- 1 small red onion, thinly sliced
- 2 tablespoons olive oil
- 2 tablespoons lemon juice
- ¼ cup chopped parsley
- A pinch of salt and black pepper

Directions:

1.In a salad bowl, mix the cucumbers with the avocados, onion, oil, lemon juice, parsley, salt, and pepper. Serve for breakfast.

Nutrition: calories 120, fat 2, fiber 2, carbs 3, protein 4

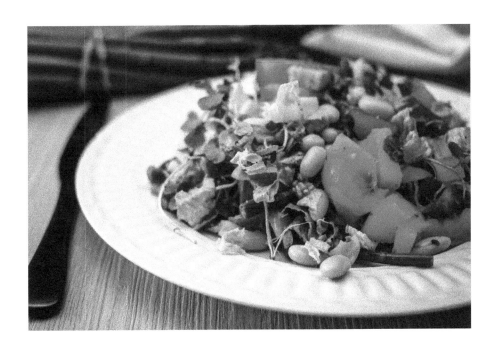

9 781802 698275